How To Get The Most Out Of Juicing

321 Great Tips For Juicing The Right Way

ADAM COLTON

Published by BizMove
www.bizmove.com

321 Great Tips For Juicing The Right Way

Juice is one of the most popular drinks in the world. Every year, customers spend millions of dollars on buying canned or bottled juice from the supermarket. Obviously, these people are unaware of the better quality and price that you get when you begin juicing fruits and vegetables yourself. This book contains tips and tricks for anything relating to juicing.

1. If you are worried about getting enough protein in your diet, add spinach and broccoli to your juices. Both of these vegetables provide enough vegetable protein for the short-term to satisfy your body's needs. Most people get more than enough protein in their daily diet, and don't need to worry about adding protein sources such as soy to their juice.

2. To get more variety in taste from your juicer, mix up the varieties of fruits and vegetables you put in your juicer and the variety of flavors will grow significantly. Try mixing orange, banana and pineapple for a tasty tropical treat or mix grape and cranberry for more antioxidants. These

homemade juices are healthier and easier to make then those sugar-filled, store bought juices.

3. In clue the whole fruit whenever you can to increase the nutritional punch of the juice you're making. Apple skin, for example, holds more nutrients than all of the flesh combined! Some peels won't taste good, like oranges, but you could zest the outside which contains a ton of flavor.

4. When it comes to juicing, one thing that you want to keep in mind is that you will want to keep your juicer out and in sight at all times. This is important to ensure that you use it on a regular basis and that it does not become one of those items that gets stored away in the back of your cupboard.

5. When it comes to juicing, one thing that you want to keep in mind is that you should build your entire healthy lifestyle around it. This is important because it is an enjoyable way to get your body all of the nutrients that it needs and with a healthy diet, you will be motivated to make healthy choices in other areas of your life.

6. Did you know that vegetable juice helps to keep blood sugar levels from spiking? It's true! It

doesn't have a lot of sugar, and half as many calories as fruit juice. It also helps you feel full for a long time, curbing any snacking cravings you might have. Try a mix of carrot and parsley to end any temptations!

7. Juicing is a great way to get delicious, fresh juice and also many important nutrients. If you need to store the juice you have made, be sure to store it in an airtight container that is opaque. It is important to be sure that there is no extra air in the container and that the juice is stored for no more than twenty four hours.

8. In regards to juicing, it is important to consider the fact that it does remove the fiber intake that you would have gotten from eating the fruit outright. Be sure to obtain fiber in other ways if you had been relying on your fruits and vegetables as your main source.

9. A great juicing tip is to not be alarmed if you see any pulp in your juice. Not only is it normal for pulp to be in juice, it enhances the flavor and also provides more nutrition. If you want the most nutrition out of your juice, keep the pulp.

10. Doing a meal plan every week can save you tons of money on your juicing needs. For example, if

you plan to use broccoli every day in juices and in meals, you can buy more of it, especially if it's on sale this week! In fact, check flyers and include sales items as often as possible for the biggest budget savings. Many stores have them online for ease of use.

11. In regards to juicing, it is important to consider the fact that certain fruits high in sugar can have a negative impact on your dental health. This is important to consider because while it may have other positive health benefits, you do not want cavities. Be sure to brush your teeth regularly after consuming drinks high in sugar.

12. A great juicing tip is to not overdo it if you're relatively new to juicing. Our bodies need time to adjust to changes. If you start drinking super healthy green juices, you might find yourself making several trips to the bathroom every day. Moderation is the key when it comes to juicing.

13. Juicing is a great way to treat acne from the inside out. Try including foods like apricots, carrots, grapefruit, mango, pumpkin, strawberries, or watercress, as they all include the best vitamins and nutrients to battle the causes of pimples. They also taste great, so it's a far

more enjoyable way to treat your skin than smelly chemical creams.

14. To gain the most benefits from making your own juice at home, make it a habit. Consume juice daily by replacing a daily snack with fruit and vegetable juice. Make sure you drink your juice no later than 20 minutes after you make it for the best health benefits.

15. Juicing is an awesome way to deal with anaemia as opposed to spending money on over-the-counter treatments which tend not to be easily digested. Include apricots, cherries, dandelion leaves, grapefruit, kiwi, lemons, strawberries and watercress to help increase your iron levels in a healthy, natural way. This will bring healthy benefits to all of your body, so enjoy the results!

16. Stop buying expensive vitamins in you are committed to a regular juicing diet. Vitamin pills are great, but they do not provide the same value as fresh juice. The health benefits start to diminish after the item has been processed so you will get better benefits from a fresh glass of juice.

17. In conclusion, you want to familiarize yourself with juicing and make sure that it is something

you want to involve yourself in, before committing to it financially. The advice provided here in this article should be more than enough to help you form your own opinions and get started.

18. If you're going to be making juice with dark, leafy greens, throw some cucumber into the mix. Some leafy greens do not taste good. Cucumber will overpower this and make the drink tastier. Cucumber, especially unpeeled cucumber, contains a variety of healthy nutrients.

19. Look into getting a system for vacuum sealing your jars if you are planning on making larger quantities of juice at the same time. Being able to fully vacuum seal your container means you will be able to store it for much longer periods of time without suffering a loss in quality or health benefits.

20. Wheat grass is only usable by us when it has been juiced. We physically can't process the fibers when it is in plant form. Learning to enjoy wheat grass will provide your body with benefits from nourishing your kidneys, providing vitalization to your skin and body, and removing toxic metals from your body's cells.

21. If you want to be successful at juicing in order to maintain a healthier lifestyle, then be sure to keep your juicing machine on your counter or in sight all the time. If you keep a certain area designated as the "juicing area," then you will be more likely to use it as it is intended.

22. Leaving some seeds in your juicer is perfectly fine! Larger seeds such as cherry pits or sometimes citrus seeds might actually damage your juicer, though, so it's best to consider the size and firmness of the seeds in the items you're juicing before throwing them in whole with reckless abandon!

23. When you have your juicer assembled, prepare the fruits or vegetables quickly so you will not have to stop and start during the juicing process. Look at juicing as if you were making a meal. Having everything on hand before you begin to cook is always easier than trying to find what you need during the process!

24. When it comes to juicing, one thing that you want to keep in mind is to be sure that you stay away from certain types of dry or squishy products when buying your ingredients. This is important because certain fruits and vegetables

such as bananas and squash are just simply not suited for juicing.

25. Using wheat-grass in your juice is an excellent way to add a ton of tasty nutrients to the final product. Start with a little bit and increase how much you push through the machine until it's all fed into the juicer. Follow with a hard fruit or vegetable to clean out the machine.

26. When it comes to juicing, one thing that you want to keep in mind is that when purchasing a juicer you will want to get a dual gear juicer. This is important, because with the extraction process used by this type of juicer, the most amount of enzymes and nutrients are retained.

27. When it comes to juicing, one thing that you want to keep in mind is the fact that certain juicers can be extremely loud. This is important to consider if you make your juice at odd times or if you live in apartment style housing. Be sure to read reviews to see which juicers are quieter.

28. Want to know another way that juicing will save you money? You'll be able to skip the expensive anti-wrinkle and deep moisturizing skin treatments you've been buying at the department store! Juicing fruits and vegetables leads to

healthier, better looking skin as they are full of moisturizing compounds. The anti-oxidants found in many produce items also can slow down the aging of skin itself.

29. Sugar is bad for your teeth, and so is chewing on sugar cane, but did you know that sugar cane JUICE is actually GOOD for your teeth? Add it to any vegetable juice you'd like sweetened and it can help prevent tooth decay while tasting absolutely great in the resulting product!

30. When it comes to juicing, one thing that you want to keep in mind is the fact that you do not need to depend on multivitamins or other supplements as much when using your juicer on a regular basis. This is beneficial because it will help you financially and give you a fun and tasty way to obtain the same nutrients.

31. Some people claim that mixing fruit and vegetables in your juice leads to indigestion as the enzymes required to break down fruit are very different than those to break down vegetables. I, personally, have never had a problem, but if you find you have any tummy upset after drinking a mixed juice then you should probably stick to one or the other.

32. In regards to juicing, it is important to consider the fact that it is best to drink your home made juice at room temperature. This is important to consider because this temperature provides the best environment for adequate consumption of nutrients into your body. Always store your juice in a cool environment, however.

33. Think about drinking your juice just before a meal to help you feel full faster, limiting your intake of solid food. The juice will digest quickly, giving you a boost in energy and providing you with the servings of fruit and vegetables you require. You'll end up eating less solid food, so try to include whole grains as it will increase your fiber intake.

34. In regards to juicing, it is important to consider the benefits that coconut can provide to your juice. Coconut is a natural way to enhance the sweetness and overall flavor of your juice. Even if you do not care for the taste of coconut, you can try adding small amounts to give you good results.

35. Juicing is a great way to remain healthy and have fun creating your own concoctions. Using fresh fruits and vegetables to create your own juice can ensure that you are getting the vitamins and

nutrients you want or need without all the sugar or preservatives. This is also a way to save a lot of money on juice!

36. If you are worried about getting enough protein in your diet, add spinach and broccoli to your juices. Both of these vegetables provide enough vegetable protein for the short-term to satisfy your body's needs. Most people get more than enough protein in their daily diet, and don't need to worry about adding protein sources such as soy to their juice.

37. Adding vegetables to your juice is a wonderful idea for getting more nutrients. Any type of leafy green is going to give you a stronger flavor; if you want to mask the taste of the veggies, try using cucumbers. You don't even need to peel them before putting them through your juicer, and they won't overpower the taste.

38. Getting kids to get the vitamins that are in vegetables, is not as difficult if you juice. Juicing has come a long way in a very short amount of time. You can juice many fruits and vegetables together to create a delicious juice cocktail that your kids will surely enjoy. You will enjoy it, too, because you know they are getting the vitamins

and minerals that they need, so they will be strong and healthy.

39. Do not assault your taste buds with crazy blends right away. Take it slow with your flavor blends and stick to what you know you will like at first. Then begin to incorporate items that you do not normally consume as juice, such as spinach or other leafy vegetables. This will prevent you from ruining the pleasure of juicing because you got a bad taste in your mouth.

40. One of the best ways to increase your nutrient intake is to make your own juice. Juicing fresh fruits and vegetables can not only be healthy, but quite tasty. Start with your favorite vegetables and then make the move to fruits. You will never want bottled juice again.

41. Let color be your guide for variety. You will want to keep your juicing varied so as to not get bored with it. Incorporate a variety of colors in your fruits and vegetables as a sort of juicing palette from which to create. Just remember to know the nutrient content from each source and enjoy the rainbow.

42. Get the best juicer for your money. Quality in juicers is no laughing matter. Target a juicer that

you can afford of course, but also look for reviews on the juicer. You will want a juicer that is quiet, highly efficient and also easy to clean. Having a quality juicer will make juicing much more enjoyable in the long run.

43. Skip a water fast and instead, engage in a vegetable juice fast! It supplies all of the nutrients and vitamins you need, without any fat and not a ton of calories. It can also help clear out toxins in your body, especially if you use wheatgrass or ginger in your recipes.

44. When it comes to juicing, one thing that you want to keep in mind is that the best way to keep pulp from your juice is through a coffee filter. This is good to keep in mind because not only are they cheap but they do a great job!

45. Jerusalem artichokes are an excellent addition to the juice you make as they will kill any craving your sweet tooth throws at you! They aren't the most flavorful food, though, so add other items like lemon juice and carrot to make a drink that you'll enjoy and will keep you healthy.

46. Buying fresh, organic produce for juicing doesn't have to cost you an arm and a leg. Buying fruit on sale can provide you with a base for which to

plan your week's juices on! For example, if apples are on sale you should choose other ingredients that go well with apples, like ginger or oranges. If berries are out of season and expensive, skip them entirely.

47. Juicing and coupon use can go hand in hand, as long as you know what you're doing. There are many coupons available for fruit, in fact I have some here right now for lemons and bananas. Use them when the fruit is on sale to increase your discount and keep as much money in your pocket as possible.

48. Getting older is a fact of life. It is also one that we try to deny and cover up. Don't let yourself get stuck in an era that was considered your prime. Holding on to clothing and make up styles from a particular decade, won't keep you that age indefinitely. It just makes you look desperate.

49. A great juicing tip is to make sure you store your juice in a way so that it doesn't lose any of its nutritional value. A good way to do this is to be absolutely sure that there is no extra air space in your juice container.

50. It's a great idea to plan out your meals for the week, including your juices. You can figure out which vegetables you'll eat when, whether it be solid or juiced, so you know exactly how much of everything you'll need to buy. This will also save you money as you can buy in bulk for multiple meals.

51. Be aware that wheat-grass is actually gluten free so if you know someone or if you suffer from a gluten intolerance you are free to use wheat grass in your juicing. The benefits from wheat grass are incredible so give it a shot and start incorporating it into your juicing endeavors.

52. Be consistent and do a little juicing everyday. The more you do, the more you'll want to juice and gradually, you'll make juicing a bigger part of your day. If you make juicing an infrequent occurrence, not only will you get less nutritional benefit but you'll also lose the will to keep going.

53. Make sure you always have the ingredients you need for juicing. Also, make them as visible as possible in your refrigerator or on the counter. If you forget they're there you might not use them, leading them to spoil and end up thrown out. Keep your turnover high so you're using the freshest ingredients possible.

54. The best time to fire up your juicer is a half hour before any meal. Drink the fresh juice on an empty stomach. Drinking juice on an empty stomach is helpful to absorb the most nutrients quickly and effectively. Fruit juices should be consumed in the mornings because digestive energy is the lowest in the mornings.

55. When juicing, it's very important to drink the juice as soon as possible while it is fresh. This will ensure that you are receiving the maximum benefits. Some nutrients begin to be destroyed right away through oxidation. If drinking immediately is impossible, store the juice in an airtight container and drink within 24 hours.

56. If you are going to increase the amount of natural nutrients you take in by juicing regularly, be prepared to go through a detox phase. If your diet consists of a high level of processed foods, your body will have to go through an adjustment phase when it is faced with handling a large influx of wholesome nutrients.

57. When it comes to juicing, one thing that you want to keep in mind is that when you are first starting out it is a good idea to keep your juices

simple. This is important to figure out the basics and what tastes good so you can build on them.

58. Skip a water fast and instead, engage in a vegetable juice fast! It supplies all of the nutrients and vitamins you need, without any fat and not a ton of calories. It can also help clear out toxins in your body, especially if you use wheatgrass or ginger in your recipes.

59. Wonder why your skin is turning a bit yellow now that you've started juicing? Don't worry, you aren't developing jaundice! Carrot juice can lend the skin a slight orange tint which will give you a sunny glow, attesting to your new healthy lifestyle. It's not a horrible skin condition after all!

60. Studies have shown that the optimal intake of fruit and vegetables in a day is 8 or 9 servings per day. Most people are lucky to even get 2 to 3, but by juicing you can meet your minimums easily and tastily! Make sure that the bulk of the servings, preferably 5 to 6, are vegetables.

61. Certain juices are very potent, so contact your pediatrician before giving any juice to a small child. Some fruits can cause diarrhea in large doses, for example, so while they just keep you

regular they could instead keep your child regularly in the bathroom! If you can't get to the doctor any time soon, stick to juice that is typically sold with kids in mind, like apple and orange.

62. In regards to juicing, it is important to know that you might experience a slight change in the color of your skin when consuming a lot of carrot juice. This is only temporary and will cause no harm to you.

63. In regards to juicing, it is important to consider the fact that it does remove the fiber intake that you would have gotten from eating the fruit outright. Be sure to obtain fiber in other ways if you had been relying on your fruits and vegetables as your main source.

64. A great juicing tip is to - know how thin or thick - you want your juice to be. Juicing bananas or avocados for example, will make a puree, which might be way too thick for what you want. Putting these foods in the blender first, will help thin them out.

65. When you get really serious about juicing you may wish to purchase a smaller second fridge just for your produce. This will leave you room in

your main fridge for solid foods and condiments. If you get really serious, you may be able to move your solid foods to the smaller fridge! That's probably a healthier way to live.

66. When using juicing as part of your weight loss program, make sure you're doing it at a time that works best for you. If you find you're rushing or stressed while creating your juices then you're likely to quit. Work it into your life as best you can, so if you can only do it every other day, it's better than nothing!

67. Do not make your juice too complicated. Select two or three vegetables, add a little apple to make it sweeter and you will create a delicious and nutritious juice. Whether you are using fruits or vegetables, making your drink too complicated means that it will not taste as good, it takes more work to produce, and so you will not enjoy it as much.

68. At the beginning of a juicing program, make juices out of fruits that you already enjoy eating. This will ensure that you enjoy the juice while still receiving some health benefits. If you start juicing using fruits you've never tried before, you may not like the juice and you're unlikely to

continue making them, meaning you won't gain any benefits.

69. Make sure to let your juicer rest and clean out extra pulp if you are making a large batch of juice, especially when you are using harder fruits. Juicers tend to be expensive, and you do not want to burn your juicer out by overworking it or clogging the juicer.

70. Look into juicers that use the masticating process instead of the centrifuge process for extraction. The masticating way of juicing preserves many more nutrients than the centrifuge, the reduction of heat produced during the process. A centrifuge juicer can still be a great value just do your homework first.

71. If storing your juice, use only air tight containers to avoid the damage from oxidation. Refrigerate your juice and as a little helper, add in just a little bit of lemon juice to help keep your juice as fresh as possible. Following these steps should lead you to still have tasty, healthy juice even hours after you did the juicing.

72. Do not forget to remove hard pits from fruits like peaches and cherries before sending them down the juicer. These pits can destroy your

juicers blades turning your happy purchase into a giant paperweight. Don't get into such a flow in your juicing that you forget to make the fruits safe for juicing.

73. When making home-made juice, it's by far the best to drink it fresh. If you must store it, use an opaque, airtight container with no air inside. To remove air, you can either add filtered water or use a food saver to suck out the excess air. Don't store fresh juice for more than 24 hours, even under these conditions.

74. Wash your juicing equipment immediately after you have finished juicing. You can actually stain your juice jugs, as well as the blades with vegetable and fruit juice.

75. Leaving a piece of fruit on the counter to rot will show you what will happen to your body if you stop eating healthy raw foods. That is exactly what happens to your organs when you eat nothing but processed garbage! If you're feeling unmotivated, look at that fruit and remember why you've chosen to juice.

76. Try not to confuse your body with your juice blends. Vegetables and fruits are digested differently by your body. Stick to juice blends

that are all fruit or all veggie when possible. Carrot is a great vegetable to sweeten the veggie mixes or use apple sparingly in the mix when dealing with greens.

77. Buy a juicer that does NOT heat up any parts near the items being juiced. The heat can cause the juice to begin oxidation, leading to a breakdown of the nutrients in it. Choose a juicer that says specifically that the parts touching the juice will remain cool throughout the juicing process.

78. When it comes to juicing, one thing that you want to keep in mind, is that you need to prepare yourself mentally and financially, for investing a lot of money into a quality juicer. This is important to consider and save for because quality juicers can cost upwards of $1500.

79. The task of picking the best juicer for your needs can be daunting. You need to consider how much juicing you plan to do. A standard machine will be great if you juice every now and then. An advanced machine will be best if you plan to juice every day.

80. When it comes to juicing, one thing that you want to keep in mind is the fact that despite the

time and money that you are losing by making your own juice, you will find that it most likely tastes better than store bought juice. This is important to give you a good reason to keep on juicing and influence others to do the same.

81. When it comes to juicing, one thing that you want to keep in mind is that not all fruits taste good when combined with each other. This is important to consider in terms of taste and overall enjoyment of your juice. Probably the most difficult fruit to mix would be certain types of melon.

82. Don't juice fruits that don't have a higher water content, such as bananas and avocados. They'll do better in a blender. In a juicer, they will just cause friction and interfere with the juicing of the other fruits that you put in. You don't want to break your juicer, in the process.

83. If you don't like the taste of certain vegetables that you should be eating for their nutritional benefit, try mixing them with fruit or vegetables you do like! Use only one disliked vegetable in a recipe and the flavors of the others that you do enjoy will overwhelm your taste buds so you don't even notice it!

84. If receiving nutrition in an easy way is a reason for trying out juicing, it is a good idea for you to learn what vitamins and minerals are in the fruit or vegetables that you would be using. This way, you will be able to pick the right produce for the nutrition that you want to receive.

85. One of the great advantages to drinking natural juiced drinks daily is that it helps cure a variety of different ailments. For example, cabbage juice helps heal different types of ulcers. For this, it is necessary to consult a medical professional first.

86. Getting into juicing can not only make you healthier, but can be a fun way to create delicious and nutritious drinks for you and your family. If you can get yourself a juicer, you can reap the benefits of a healthier way to drink juice. Plus, you'll know it wasn't made in a factory somewhere. Unless you have a juicer in a factory you work at!

87. Bananas and papayas do not seem to do well in a juicer. You can still use them with juice, but it is best to stick them in a blender. They are very thick, and tend to work better when making fruit smoothies or any type of frozen dessert that you make.

88. The best place to find the freshest produce for juicing at great prices is at a local farmer's market. Often, they are held once a week during the summer and fall months, and you'll find everything sold on a farm, including meat, eggs, dairy, baked goods, canned goods, and TONS of fresh fruit and vegetables!

89. When it comes to juicing, one thing that you want to keep in mind is that you will want to make sure that you purchase all of your fruits and vegetables from local farmers markets. Local farmers markets often will have a greater selection and lower prices than normal grocery stores.

90. When it comes to juicing, one thing that you want to keep in mind is that you want to ensure that all of the fruits and vegetables that you purchase are cleaned as well as possible. This is important for health reasons as well as making sure that there are no outside factors that effect the taste of your juice.

91. When it comes to juicing, one thing that you want to keep in mind is that when you are dealing with greens such as lettuce, it is best to stack it up in a dense pile before putting it in your juicer. This is important because you will

get the most amount of juice and nutrients this way.

92. When it comes to juicing, one thing to remember is the only way for the body to process wheat grass is by juicing it. This is important, because you are creating a way to introduce important ingredients into your body that you could not have done otherwise.

93. When juicing soft fruits such as melons, peaches and strawberries it is good to know that the resulting juice will be thicker as opposed to juicing hard fruits such as apples. A good way to have great juice is combining both of these juices. This will create balance and will result in a much better texture.

94. In regards to juicing, it is important to consider the fact that juices can actually work to prevent cancer in your body. The benefit from this is obvious and it does so through the maintenance of proper pH levels. Many types of produce also work to rid the body of toxins.

95. Maintaining blood sugar levels helps to curb hunger, so including carrot juice in your creations can help you keep healthy and eat less. Carrots do have more sugar in them than many

other vegetables, but the fact that they don't cause a spike in blood glucose means that you can overlook that and drink them up!

96. Jerusalem artichokes are an excellent addition to the juice you make as they will kill any craving your sweet tooth throws at you! They aren't the most flavorful food, though, so add other items like lemon juice and carrot to make a drink that you'll enjoy and will keep you healthy.

97. In regards to juicing, it is important to consider consulting with a doctor if you are currently pregnant or planning on getting pregnant in the near future. This is important because you want to make sure that the potentially powerful effects of consuming homemade juice will be beneficial to your baby.

98. Juicing and coupon use can go hand in hand, as long as you know what you're doing. There are many coupons available for fruit, in fact I have some here right now for lemons and bananas. Use them when the fruit is on sale to increase your discount and keep as much money in your pocket as possible.

99. A great juicing tip that can help extend the life of your juicer, is to only use your juice on a hard

surface. By using your juicer on a hard surface you'll insure that there won't be any vibrations. Vibrations, no matter how small, can damage your juicer over time.

100.   Have you ever been happy to be sick? I haven't either, but a case of bronchitis can be aided by some tasty juices which will make you a lot happier than any medicine that you'd be prescribed! Try grape, lemon, onion, and orange juice to soothe the pain and help kill off the nasty germs that are making you sick.

101.   Green juices are jammed packed with vitamins and minerals. There is some misinformation out there about the taste of the green juices though. This does not have to be true all the time. You can juice additional ingredients to improve the taste. For instance, to make the juice a little sour, add limes; to make it taste sweeter, add apples.

102.   A good juicing tip is to make sure you aren't adding in any fruits or vegetables that have gone bad. A lot of people make the mistake of throwing in produce that's overripe because they don't want to be wasteful. This can spoil your juice and make it less nutritional.

103.   Drink your juice soon after making it if you are looking to benefit from the health benefits. Juice starts to lose its benefits as soon as it comes out of the fruit or veggie. The longer you let it sit, the more it will lose, so go ahead and drink it as soon as possible to be able to let your body enjoy all the nutrients.

104.   When making carrot juice, make absolutely sure to get fresh, healthy carrots. Signs of old carrots are rubberiness, limpness, wilted tops, and excessive cracking. Look for carrots that have a full color, are firm to the touch, and have green, leafy tops. These carrots will produce the freshest, sweetest juice.

105.   Store all your fruits and vegetables in the refrigerator, especially in the summertime. Juicing depends on fresh produce and leaving them out starts the process of decay more quickly. Keep your produce nice and cool until you eat it so that you can preserve as many vitamins as you can.

106.   Wash your juicing equipment immediately after you have finished juicing. In addition, some vegetables and fruits will stain the juicer if it sits too long before cleaning.

107.   If you want to improve your nutrition, give juicing a try. Juicing makes it easy to get all of your daily recommended servings of fruits and vegetables. While you will miss out on the fiber these foods provide, you will get all of the vitamins and minerals, and juice tastes great too!

108.   Let color be your guide for variety. You will want to keep your juicing varied so as to not get bored with it. Incorporate a variety of colors in your fruits and vegetables as a sort of juicing palette from which to create. Just remember to know the nutrient content from each source and enjoy the rainbow.

109.   Remember that vegetable and fruit remnants left on a juicer after juicing have the potential to grow mold quickly. Cleaning it quickly helps stop the growth of mold. Dismantle the juicer clean the parts and rinse with water until clean. If you must use a detergent use one that is very mild.

110.   You know the health benefits of juicing but you need a juicer. Researching the different types of juicers will help you decide which machine will meet your needs. There are masticating juicers, centrifugal juicers and manual press juicers. These juicers complete the process

differently but the end result is a tasty glass of juice.

111.   When it comes to juicing, one thing that you want to keep in mind is that you will want to make sure that you purchase all of your fruits and vegetables from local farmers markets. Local farmers markets often will have a greater selection and lower prices than normal grocery stores.

112.   When it comes to juicing, one thing that you want to keep in mind is to be sure that you stay away from certain types of dry or squishy products when buying your ingredients. This is important because certain fruits and vegetables such as bananas and squash are just simply not suited for juicing.

113.   When it comes to juicing, it can be easy to lose enthusiasm for it. However, if you can share ideas about juicing with a personal friend or on a forum of some kind, you will find it easier to get inspired with new ideas. This sort of dialogue can also remind you of the wonderful health benefits that come from consuming a wide variety of juiced fruits and vegetables.

114.   Did you know that juice can help you supress your appetite? Having a glass of vegetable juice will provide you with a ton of nutrients, but it will also fill your stomach and make your body think that you've just engaged in a heavy meal. The fiber in vegetables keep you feeling full for a long time, curbing your temptation to eat.

115.   When it comes to juicing, one thing that you want to keep in mind is that when you are first starting out it is a good idea to keep your juices simple. This is important to figure out the basics and what tastes good so you can build on them.

116.   When it comes to juicing, one thing that you want to keep in mind is the fact that wheat grass is not only an extremely powerful tasting ingredient but it also provides many nutrients. This is important because you want to introduce this into your juices, but you need to be careful to not use too much due to its overpowering taste.

117.   In regards to juicing, it is important to consider the fact that it is best to drink your home made juice at room temperature. This is important to consider because this temperature provides the best environment for adequate

consumption of nutrients into your body. Always store your juice in a cool environment, however.

118.   In regards to juicing, it is important to consider adding ginger to your juice. This is beneficial not only because it can add some good spice to it, but it also has its own benefits of being a natural way to combat having an upset stomach or experiencing nauseousness.

119.   The best place to get your herbs, vegetables, and fruit is from your garden. Planting and tending to them will also give you exercise! If you live in an apartment or condo, grow some plants on your balcony. If you don't have a balcony you can find local co-op gardens which will permit you to take some of their produce in return for pitching in and working for a few hours a week.

120.   If you want your juice to be a certain texture or thickness, know that the softer the fruit is, the thicker the juice will be. The meat of softer fruits breaks up easily to make a thick nectar. Make sure to add some harder fruits, such as apples and pears, for a thinner juice.

121.   Keep all the tools you use in juicing, like your cutting board, knives, measuring cups,

juicer, etc. together in their own place so you always know where they are. The one reason you won't continue juicing is because you're not keeping your things organized, leaving you feeling frustrated and overwhelmed.

122.　Are you diabetic? Juicing can still be for you! You can juice so many different items that you'll always be able to have a selection that does not contain too many carbohydrates or a large dose of sugar. You can also include milk or yogurt in your drink to up your dairy intake.

123.　Try adding chopped ice to your juice to make it a cool treat in the summer! It's like drinking a smoothie while actually knowing what ingredients are in it and where they came from (and how clean they were when they went into the juicer!) What a tasty way to chill out.

124.　When juicing for your health you should drink the juice as soon as it's made. Refrigerating the juice or leaving it on the counter will allow it to lose nutrients as they break down within the juice. Drinking it immediately will be just like eating all those fresh ingredients whole!

125.　Using wheat-grass in your juice is an excellent way to add a ton of tasty nutrients to the final product. Start with a little bit and increase how much you push through the machine until it's all fed into the juicer. Follow with a hard fruit or vegetable to clean out the machine.

126.   When it comes to juicing, one thing that you want to keep in mind is that sometimes you may need to add in artificial flavors to attain a certain taste that you desire. This is important because while you may feel as though you are cheating, there are some flavors that are just not reasonable to obtain from normal juicing procedures.

127.   Make sure you drink your juices as soon as you make them. Time is important for juicing because the valuable nutrients will become oxidized when exposed to the air. So you always want to drink your juices quickly. If, for some reason you can't, then try to store the juice in an air-tight container to minimize oxidation.

128.   If receiving nutrition in an easy way is a reason for trying out juicing, it is a good idea for you to learn what vitamins and minerals are in the fruit or vegetables that you would be using. This way, you will be able to pick the right

produce for the nutrition that you want to receive.

129.   To get the most nutrition from your juices, be sure to drink them when they are fresh. After juicing, fruits and vegetables are vulnerable to oxidation which will destroy their nutrients. If you have to store your juices for some reason, use air tight containers to reduce the amount of oxidation that will happen.

130.   Everyone knows vegetable and fruit juice is healthy, but did you know that juices containing phytochemicals are able to reduce the amount of carcinogens found in your body? Use as many of these phytochemical-rich foods as you can.

131.   If you want to have a juice that tastes like a commercial smoothie, add some vanilla! Skip the extract and go for the real thing - scrape a vanilla pod and enjoy the smooth, creamy flavor it imparts on the final product. If you really want to fulfill the smoothie experience, add a little non-fat, unsweetened yogurt to your drink.

132.   The pith on citrus fruit, the white part between the skin and the pulp, is full of nutrients that are fabulous for you, so make sure to pull it out of the fruit with the pulp when you're

juicing. It has bio-flavonoids and tons of vitamin C, so bulk up on it during flu season!

133.　When you're creating juices for healthy benefits, you should use at least half or two-thirds dark green vegetables, like kale, chard, broccoli, or parsley. Also use herbs juices including mint, rosemary, and basil. Look for dessert recipes online to see great fruit and herb combinations you might like!

134.　One of the secrets to aging, is knowing your limits. As we get older, certain things become more difficult or inappropriate for us. Rather than trying to hold on to these things, we need to let go and allow ourselves to see that though we have gotten older, we have entered into a new and exciting time of life. Embrace where you are on your journey.

135.　You know juicing is tasty and healthy but you also need to know how to take care of your machine. Always clean the juicer immediately using it so particles do not get hard. Take the machine apart as instructed and rinse completely or put in your dishwasher. Clean the screen with a vegetable brush.

136.   A great juicing tip is to make sure you store your juice in a way so that it doesn't lose any of its nutritional value. A good way to do this is to be absolutely sure that there is no extra air space in your juice container.

137.   A masticating juicer is something you want to use. These juicers have a more gentle method of extracting juice, which helps the liquid maintain more of its nutrients. Masticating juicers also produce juice more suitable for storage.

138.   Don't forget to wash your produce prior to juicing, and use organic products where possible. So many people seem to think that since it's going to turn into juice, they don't need to wash their fruits and veggies. Just because it's liquid, doesn't mean the chemicals present on the peels are going to go away. Clean your fruits and vegetables thoroughly before juicing.

139.   When starting to juice it's better to start slow. Use flavors you already know you like and don't try new things until you know you're ready. Start by mixing new flavors, like wheat grass, with fruit you've already been drinking. Soon enough you'll be able to move on to pro recipes!

140.   Leaving a piece of fruit on the counter to rot will show you what will happen to your body if you stop eating healthy raw foods. That is exactly what happens to your organs when you eat nothing but processed garbage! If you're feeling unmotivated, look at that fruit and remember why you've chosen to juice.

141.   If you find that your juicer becomes oily after juicing citrus fruits such as oranges, limes, lemons and grapefruits you will have to clean the juicer with a mild detergent to get the oily feeling off. This is residue left behind from the citrus must be cleansed well to avoid complications with mold.

142.   Always drink your juice right away after you have put it through the juicer! This is when the juice is most potent and has the most nutritional value. If you cannot get to it right away, get to the juice and drink it as soon as possible. Do not make a large amount of juice to store.

143.   If you're feeling bloated or retaining water, put the right ingredients into your juice to help flush you out! Celery, cranberry, cucumber, and watermelon are all recommended to help your system let the water go, and they also hold many

nutrients, vitamins, and other healthy benefits that are vital to good health.

144.   To get the most nutrition from your juices, be sure to drink them when they are fresh. After juicing, fruits and vegetables are vulnerable to oxidation which will destroy their nutrients. If you have to store your juices for some reason, use air tight containers to reduce the amount of oxidation that will happen.

145.   In regards to juicing, it is important to consider adding ginger to your juice. This is beneficial not only because it can add some good spice to it, but it also has its own benefits of being a natural way to combat having an upset stomach or experiencing nauseousness.

146.   In regards to juicing, it is important to consider the fact that while this will provide many benefits to your health and overall well being, it is not the only solution. This is critical because if you are not taking care of your body in other ways, you may diminish or eliminate the effects you are receiving from consuming your home made juices.

147.   People who want to juice but who have acid reflux, problems with candida like thrush,

diabetes, or intestinal issues should avoid putting too much fruit in their recipes. Green items like kale, parsley, chard, and broccoli will change the pH of the body to a more healthy level, lowering your pH and blood sugar.

148.   Juicing may sound scary if you have problems with acidity like heartburn, but there are many fruit and vegetables which will actually combat the acid and help heal your gastrointestinal tract. They include beets, carrots, grapes, oranges, peaches, spinach and tomatoes. Try to drink at least 32 ounces of these items a day for maximum health benefits.

149.   If your blood pressure is high, it's time to buy a juicer! Vegetables and fruit carry so many health benefits, and increasing your intake will not only help you battle blood pressure, but it's likely to cause weight loss and replace sodium-rich foods you might not eat otherwise. Choose cucumber, garlic, lemon, parsley or pear for the biggest blood pressure regulation benefits.

150.   A good juicing tip is to make sure you clean your juicer right after you use it. Cleaning your juicer right after use will prevent particles from hardening, which will make the juicer much

easier to clean. You'll save a lot of time and energy by doing this.

151.   Are you tired of the same old smoothies? You can find a lot of recipes in a cookbook at your local bookstore or on the Internet. Don't just make the same juice each day, instead find new and exciting recipes to try.

152.   You should explore the internet for recipes and find the ones that not only sound good to you, but that have comments from other users endorsing the recipe. This will ensure that you do not waste your valuable time and produce on a drink that you do not enjoy. In time you will be able to create your own recipes.

153.   Instead of pulling out your juicer every time you want fresh juice, make extra and store it. In order to properly store juice you will want to put it in a opaque, airtight container and make sure that there is no extra air space in that container. Try using distilled water to make up the extra space.

154.   Crumple up leafy greens, such as spinach, into tight balls before putting them in your juicer. Your juicer is primarily designed to deal with solid fruits and vegetables, not thin leaves.

You will get better results from your juicer if you simulate this effect by squashing your leafy greens before juicing.

155.   Brush your teeth as soon as possible after drinking fresh fruit juice. Fruit juice is naturally very high in sugar, in addition to containing acids that can eat away at tooth enamel. The longer these sugars and acids sit in your mouth, the worse the damage will be, so brush soon.

156.   Make sure and remove the greens from items like carrots and rhubarb. They can contain harmful chemicals that become toxic when juiced. Make sure to research all of your fruits, veggies and other items before juicing them so that you are aware of any important do's and don'ts before starting.

157.   When attempting a juice-only diet, it can be helpful to remove all processed foods from your house first. Having a box of crackers, a jar of peanut butter, or some candy bars staring you in the face while you can only have juice is an easy way to cut your diet tragically short.

158.   If you are going to store juice that you have made yourself, you need to do this correctly. Choose a container that is airtight, and add a

couple of drops of lemon juice to it before putting it into the refrigerator. Label your juice so that you remember what you are drinking, and enjoy!

159. The best place to find the freshest produce for juicing at great prices is at a local farmer's market. Often, they are held once a week during the summer and fall months, and you'll find everything sold on a farm, including meat, eggs, dairy, baked goods, canned goods, and TONS of fresh fruit and vegetables!

160. If you have any questions about juicing you can always ask online. There are many juicing groups and forums available and their members will typically have the answer, or at least know how to find it. Draw on their collective years of experience to make your experience a positive one!

161. The best time to fire up your juicer is a half hour before any meal. Drink the fresh juice on an empty stomach. Drinking juice on an empty stomach is helpful to absorb the most nutrients quickly and effectively. Fruit juices should be consumed in the mornings because digestive energy is the lowest in the mornings.

162.   When looking for a juicer to purchase, check out the additional features it provides. A masticating juicer often comes with attachments to make pasta or grind foods, which can save you money by making other foods from scratch as well. Consider the juicer an investment for your whole kitchen, and pick up a few attachments while you're out.

163.   When coming up with a combination of fruit and vegetables to juice, consider their textures to make a smooth, drinkable product. For example, soft fruits like bananas and peaches make a very thick juice. Apples and pears, on the other hand, make a very thin, watery juice. Mix the two items together to make the most enjoyable texture to drink!

164.   If you're feeling bloated or retaining water, put the right ingredients into your juice to help flush you out! Celery, cranberry, cucumber, and watermelon are all recommended to help your system let the water go, and they also hold many nutrients, vitamins, and other healthy benefits that are vital to good health.

165.   Ginger is an all-natural remedy for alleviating gastrointestinal distress. It adds some kick to the flavor of your juice as well as promotes health. It

is a great anti-inflammatory agent which can aid in healing the esophageal reaction to acid reflux, or stomach ulcers and upset.

166.   Incorporate spices into your juicing. There are a variety of spices such as cinnamon, nutmeg, garlic, ginger and others, that can can boost the flavor output of your juices. If you have flavors you want to experiment with, look for recipes online or you can look for spices that work well with fruits or vegetables. Be sure to check their health and nutrition values.

167.   Studies have shown that the optimal intake of fruit and vegetables in a day is 8 or 9 servings per day. Most people are lucky to even get 2 to 3, but by juicing you can meet your minimums easily and tastily! Make sure that the bulk of the servings, preferably 5 to 6, are vegetables.

168.   One of the great advantages to drinking natural juiced drinks daily is that it helps cure a variety of different ailments. For example, cabbage juice helps heal different types of ulcers. For this, it is necessary to consult a medical professional first.

169.   In regards to juicing, it is important to consider adding ginger to your juice. This is

beneficial not only because it can add some good spice to it, but it also has its own benefits of being a natural way to combat having an upset stomach or experiencing nauseousness.

170.   A great juicing tip that can help you save time is to start eyeballing the amount of foods you'll need to make the amount of juice you want. A pound of raw produce for instance, will typically make at least one whole cup of juice. Knowing these tricks can help you save time.

171.   Dark leafy greens benefit from the addition of a cucumber when juicing. Most leafy greens will have a strong and somewhat unpleasant flavor. Cucumber helps neutralize the bad taste of other leafy greens, and adds a nice flavor of its own. Use unpeeled cucumber for essential nutrients.

172.   Crumple up leafy greens, such as spinach, into tight balls before putting them in your juicer. Your juicer is primarily designed to deal with solid fruits and vegetables, not thin leaves. You will get better results from your juicer if you simulate this effect by squashing your leafy greens before juicing.

173.   If you are worried about getting enough protein in your diet, add spinach and broccoli to your juices. Both of these vegetables provide enough vegetable protein for the short-term to satisfy your body's needs. Most people get more than enough protein in their daily diet, and don't need to worry about adding protein sources such as soy to their juice.

174.   The biggest key in juicing is curiosity. Wanting to try new foods, things you've never even heard of before, will make your journey more tasty and exciting! Explore international produce markets to find vegetables and fruit that could change your life forever. Look online to research what vitamins and nutrients they contain.

175.   Pay close attention to which vegetables and fruits your juicer recommends. There are some fruits and vegetables that do not lend themselves well to juicing. Bananas are a great example of this, as they tend to thicken a mixture when added, which is why they are used in smoothies regularly. Blend these types of produce, as opposed to juicing, for best results.

176.   One of the best ways to increase your nutrient intake is to make your own juice. Juicing

fresh fruits and vegetables can not only be healthy, but quite tasty. Start with your favorite vegetables and then make the move to fruits. You will never want bottled juice again.

177.   Before you invest in a juicer, you should do your research. Check out buying guides online, as well as customer reviews, to choose which juicer will fit your needs, while being well respected by those who have already purchased one. A juicer is a big investment, so don't jump into it without knowing what you're doing!

178.   If you absolutely must store your juice after you make it, make sure to store it in a completely air-tight container. Letting air get at it will start a process which breaks down the nutrients in the juice, leaving a tasty but empty drink that won't provide you with the healthy benefits you were looking for in the first place.

179.   To lose weight quickly but healthfully, try juicing. Simply replace one to two meals per day with fresh green juice. There are countless recipes available online, but you can make your own by mixing a green leafy vegetable with one or two fruits. You will be getting more vitamins and minerals than the average American, but fewer calories.

180.   Start juicing with the softer items in your ingredient list and then follow them up with the harder items. This will help clear the pulp from your machine to facilitate an easier clean up later. You want to work your machine in the easiest way possible to give it a long life.

181.   When you have your juicer assembled, prepare the fruits or vegetables quickly so you will not have to stop and start during the juicing process. Look at juicing as if you were making a meal. Having everything on hand before you begin to cook is always easier than trying to find what you need during the process!

182.   When juicing, it's very important to drink the juice as soon as possible while it is fresh. This will ensure that you are receiving the maximum benefits. Some nutrients begin to be destroyed right away through oxidation. If drinking immediately is impossible, store the juice in an airtight container and drink within 24 hours.

183.   When it comes to juicing, one thing that you want to keep in mind is to be sure to listen to your body as far as how it reacts to certain types of juices. This is important to consider both in the case of positive and negative effects that your

juice can give you, ranging from allergic reactions to clarity of mind.

184.   To make sure that your juices pack the most nutritional punch, always choose organic ingredients if they are available. Organic produce has a higher nutritional content than conventionally grown produce and it also usually tastes better. You'll also avoid any possible toxic chemicals like pesticides and fertilizers that are used in conventional agriculture.

185.   It's best to avoid juicing fruits and vegetables that have a low water content. Avocados and bananas, for example, are quite dense and don't have much water in them. They will clog up your juicer and you won't get much juice out of them. If you really want to include them, blend them first and then mix them with juices from other produce.

186.   After creating your juice concoction, remember to consume it as soon as possible. To get great healthy juice, realize that some nutrients are lost when juice is made. The more time you take to drink what you've just juiced, the less nutrients you'll benefit from. Therefore, by drinking the juice as soon as it is made, you will receive the most benefit from it.

187.   Make sure to let your juicer rest and clean out extra pulp if you are making a large batch of juice, especially when you are using harder fruits. Juicers tend to be expensive, and you do not want to burn your juicer out by overworking it or clogging the juicer.

188.   Try vegetables mixed with your favorite fruits in your juicer. Many vegetables are easy to juice. They can add important vitamins and minerals to your juice as well. In addition, using vegetables can cut down on the calorie count of your juice, which in turn, makes it a better diet option.

189.   Juicing is a wonderful part of a healthy lifestyle, but you don't have to be totally strict about what you consume. You should practice excellent health choices at least two-thirds of the time. The other third allows you to go out to a restaurant, have a few potato chips, or indulge in some ice cream.

190.   Ask your friends and family if they'd like to go in on purchases in bulk at local farms with you so you can buy more and get larger discounts. Apple farms, for example, will sell you bushel after bushel for decreasing costs per

pound. Take a few cars up, load the back with apples, and share with everyone! They don't have to be juicers to enjoy fresh produce.

191.   Get adventurous with your juicing ingredients! Why not try grapefruit or add in a little ginger for some zip! Other items to try are celery, parsley, beets, bell peppers, and leafy greens! You never know what you might end up liking.

192.   Juicing is the best-tasting way to make sure you're getting all the daily servings of fruit and vegetables that you need. You can mix them together in a combination that will provide any nutrient you need, and it will taste good no matter what you include. The whole family can sip and enjoy!

193.   When it comes to juicing, one thing that you want to keep in mind is that you want to do your homework when it comes to buying a juicer. This is important to make sure that you are getting a quality product that will last you for a long time and suit all of your juicing needs.

194.   To help you decide which juicer to buy read your customer reviews of popular models before choosing the machine that is best for you. If you

are on a social network, ask your friends if they have any input on juicing machines. Word of mouth is one of the best research methods available.

195.   When figuring out your recipes and buying produce at the market, remember that approximately one pound of vegetables and fruit will lead to one cup of juice. Softer fruits will yield about as much juice as is equal to their weight as they won't lose much pulp, while harder vegetables will produce a lot of pulp and produce less juice.

196.   Reading the instruction manual that came with your juicer will help you make the best juice possible. The manual will advise you of which fruits or vegetables that may require the skin to be removed. It will also tell you which produce does not juice well, such as bananas and avocados.

197.   Make sure you drink your juices as soon as you make them. Time is important for juicing because the valuable nutrients will become oxidized when exposed to the air. So you always want to drink your juices quickly. If, for some reason you can't, then try to store the juice in an air-tight container to minimize oxidation.

198.   If you'd like to add an exotic flavor to your juice recipes, try some fresh coconut! It adds a nutty smoothness to any mixture, giving you something new and different to enjoy. Try mixing it with other exotic juices, like mango or papaya. Some like to chew on a piece of coconut while preparing their juice!

199.   A masticating juicer is the best choice for the beginner or expert alike. These juicers allow you to mill, grind, make a puree, and even create frozen deserts. These juicers offer an array of juices you can make.

200.   Cucumber juice is helpful for maintaining healthy hair and skin. There is quite a bit of silica in cucumbers. In addition, silica is beneficial for bones, muscles, tendons, and ligaments and increases the strength of connective tissue.

201.   Use cranberries! In regards to juicing, it is important to consider the benefits that cranberries can provide! As long as you care for their taste, cranberries will assist with infections of the urinary tract, as well as, the everyday benefit of helping to remove toxins from your body. Also, cranberries provide a great distinct taste that compliment many other foods.

202.   You know juicing is tasty and healthy but you also need to know how to take care of your machine. Always clean the juicer immediately using it so particles do not get hard. Take the machine apart as instructed and rinse completely or put in your dishwasher. Clean the screen with a vegetable brush.

203.   Don't let your juice sit for long before serving it. Ideally you will drink your juice as soon as you make it.

204.   Juicing is a yummy alternative to choking down broccoli or other fruits and vegetables that you just dont' like the taste of. Include as many veggies as you can into your juice by covering them up with powerful fruit flavors like apple, banana and oranges. The citrus and sweet flavors of these will have no problems masking the other flavors you are not fond of.

205.   Wheat grass is only usable by us when it has been juiced. We physically can't process the fibers when it is in plant form. Learning to enjoy wheat grass will provide your body with benefits from nourishing your kidneys, providing vitalization to your skin and body, and removing toxic metals from your body's cells.

206.   The best rule for getting into juicing is that the juicer should be out and visible all the time. This will remind you to use it, and also make it easier to use so you don't skip it because you don't want to lug it out. Keeping it in sight will also keep it in mind.

207.   One of the best ways to increase your nutrient intake is to make your own juice. Juicing fresh fruits and vegetables can not only be healthy, but quite tasty. Start with your favorite vegetables and then make the move to fruits. You will never want bottled juice again.

208.   If you're considering a raw food diet, then buying a masticating juicer is a great start! It comes with so many accessories for other food processing, like milling or pureeing, so you can use it to make all of your raw food meals. This purchase will prove to be a great start to your new healthy lifestyle!

209.   Start juicing! People begin juicing - adding freshly juiced fruits and vegetables to their diet - for a vast range of reasons. Some people juice to supplement their diet or detoxify their bodies. Some people are doing it for other health reasons. Juicing in and of itself will not cure

ailments - yet you will benefit from juicing - with extra nutrients and more energy!

210.   When it comes to juicing, one thing that you want to keep in mind is that you want to ensure that all of the fruits and vegetables that you purchase are cleaned as well as possible. This is important for health reasons as well as making sure that there are no outside factors that effect the taste of your juice.

211.   Don't juice fruits that don't have a higher water content, such as bananas and avocados. They'll do better in a blender. In a juicer, they will just cause friction and interfere with the juicing of the other fruits that you put in. You don't want to break your juicer, in the process.

212.   When it comes to juicing, one thing that you want to keep in mind is the different benefits that specific types of juice extracts will bring you. One such benefit is the fact that the juice from cabbage is a great natural way to heal stomach ulcers. This is not meant to replace other methods, but it may work great for you in addition to what you are already doing.

213.   When it comes to juicing, one thing that you want to keep in mind is the fact that you do not

need to depend on multivitamins or other supplements as much when using your juicer on a regular basis. This is beneficial because it will help you financially and give you a fun and tasty way to obtain the same nutrients.

214.   One of the great advantages to drinking natural juiced drinks daily is that it helps cure a variety of different ailments. For example, cabbage juice helps heal different types of ulcers. For this, it is necessary to consult a medical professional first.

215.   Many studies have shown that spices help to boost your metabolism along with tasting great, so include them in your juices! Hot spices used in Indian cooking are an excellent choice, so include cayenne, garam masala, cardamom, cinnamon, coriander, and allspice as often as possible to get a great boost to your fat burning system!

216.   I'd highly recommend buying a juicer with a brand name over one that you don't recognize the name of. Brand name juicers are more likely to last a long time, and will usually have a warranty or guarantee to back their claims up. Smaller companies can be fly-by-night, and you tend to get what you pay for.

217.   If you have trouble juicing ginger, use a garlic press on it first! This will release the binds within the pulp itself and allow your juicer to extract as much juice as possible from the chunk of ginger. You can also do the same for garlic you wish to use.

218.   To gain the most benefits from making your own juice at home, make it a habit. Consume juice daily by replacing a daily snack with fruit and vegetable juice. Make sure you drink your juice no later than 20 minutes after you make it for the best health benefits.

219.   A good tip to help maintain your juicer is to remove the pits from various fruits. Apple pits can ruin your juice if you forget to remove them. Other fruits such as plums and peaches have pits that should be removed as well in order to protect the juicer.

220.   A great juicing tip is to make sure you purchase a quality juicer. A great way to make sure you're getting the best juicer you can get, is to look online for juicer reviews. A lot of people will post their own product reviews, which can help you to decide if a product is right for you.

221.   Make sure you invest in the right juicer! Consider factors such as your budget, the features you are looking for, how often it will be used and how many people will use it to find the perfect juicer for your home. Choose a durable model that does not generate too much heat!

222.   Use cucumber as a great flavor disguiser when you are juicing greens. Cucumber is excellent at masking the strong flavors inherent in greens. A juice's health benefits aren't going to do you much good if you can't stand to drink it. Cucumber also has the extra added benefit of being chockfull of important vitamins and nutrients itself.

223.   When making carrot juice, make absolutely sure to get fresh, healthy carrots. Signs of old carrots are rubberiness, limpness, wilted tops, and excessive cracking. Look for carrots that have a full color, are firm to the touch, and have green, leafy tops. These carrots will produce the freshest, sweetest juice.

224.   If mixed correctly, juice can constitute your whole meal. You may be surprised to discover the volume of fruits and veggies that goes into a single glass of juice. Juice should be consumed as

a meal by itself so the nutritional value of it gets into your bloodstream much quicker.

225.   Getting kids to get the vitamins that are in vegetables, is not as difficult if you juice. Juicing has come a long way in a very short amount of time. You can juice many fruits and vegetables together to create a delicious juice cocktail that your kids will surely enjoy. You will enjoy it, too, because you know they are getting the vitamins and minerals that they need, so they will be strong and healthy.

226.   Lacking space on your cutting board for all of the ingredients you need for juicing? Try to cut everything in a manner which keeps the actual food "whole". For example, slice a carrot but don't pull the pieces apart. You can slice an apple around it's core and then stand the pieces up so it looks like it wasn't cut. This will save you space to slice the other items you need without dirtying more dishes.

227.   Be aware that citrus fruits do not always work well in all juicers. Because of the consistency of the pulp in the fruit the juicer can get clogged with the pulp or rind. If using a standard juicer, peel the fruit and cut into small

pieces; otherwise get a citrus juicer that you will use for these types of fruit specifically.

228.   Making excess juice to bottle and refrigerate is very handy, but you don't want your juice to get discolored. Nobody wants juice that was once a bright color, but now is brown or gray. One thing that can help prolong the juice is to put some fresh lemon juice in the mixture. As long as you don't add too much lemon juice, the taste will not be affected, and the juice will look fresh.

229.   There are a million-and-one recipes of items to include in your juicer. You can try a combination like apple with carrot and ginger, or celery and pear. My favorites are apple with lemon and pear, apple with cinnamon and honey, and, my daughter's favorite, banana with mango and orange. Try new ideas to find your own favorites!

230.   If you have any questions about juicing you can always ask online. There are many juicing groups and forums available and their members will typically have the answer, or at least know how to find it. Draw on their collective years of experience to make your experience a positive one!

231. It's always better to use organic fruit when making juices, but since they are pricy, you can't always get organic fruit. When using non-organic produce, there might be harmful pesticides that you don't want to put into your drinks. So, make sure you peel the fruits so you don't ingest the pesticides.

232. In regards to juicing, it is important to consider adding ginger to your juice. This is beneficial not only because it can add some good spice to it, but it also has its own benefits of being a natural way to combat having an upset stomach or experiencing nauseousness.

233. In regards to juicing, it is important to consider the fact that you are creating a natural and cheap anti-aging product. This is important to consider when you weigh the costs of a juicer and produce, against how much you may pay for other methods of staying young, such as creams or medicines.

234. If you have trouble juicing ginger, use a garlic press on it first! This will release the binds within the pulp itself and allow your juicer to extract as much juice as possible from the chunk

of ginger. You can also do the same for garlic you wish to use.

235.   Change the juices you make every day to make sure you're getting all the nutrients possible. You're also more likely to get bored of the juice you're drinking if you have the same taste over and over again, so mix it up! Go online to look up tried-and-true recipes, or ask family and friends for their advice.

236.   A great juicing tip is to not get too carried away with making sweet juices. It's nice to make juice that tastes good, but you don't want to take in too much sugar. Getting careless with making sweet juices can lead to getting in way more sugar than you want.

237.   If you can't stomach a green juice, try adding a few grapes. They go very well with the taste of dark leafy greens, and they add a sweetness which isn't overwhelming. They also contain anti-oxidants which are great for keeping your cells safe from the ravages of free radicals. Enjoy!

238.   Put all your fruit on one shelf in your refrigerator, preferably the top shelf. This way, nutrition and juicing will be the first thing on

your mind when you open your refrigerator every day. You'll also be able to keep an eye on how fresh the fruit is, and remind yourself to use it before it decays.

239.   Make sure you always have the ingredients you need for juicing. Also, make them as visible as possible in your refrigerator or on the counter. If you forget they're there you might not use them, leading them to spoil and end up thrown out. Keep your turnover high so you're using the freshest ingredients possible.

240.   Lacking space on your cutting board for all of the ingredients you need for juicing? Try to cut everything in a manner which keeps the actual food "whole". For example, slice a carrot but don't pull the pieces apart. You can slice an apple around it's core and then stand the pieces up so it looks like it wasn't cut. This will save you space to slice the other items you need without dirtying more dishes.

241.   Buy a juicer that does NOT heat up any parts near the items being juiced. The heat can cause the juice to begin oxidation, leading to a breakdown of the nutrients in it. Choose a juicer that says specifically that the parts touching the

juice will remain cool throughout the juicing process.

242.   Should you juice wheatgrass? The claims are many about it's health benefits, including the fact that it helps increase the number of red blood cells, flushes the body of toxic metals, keeps your organs in tip-top shape, and clears out your lymph system. It`s also said to increase vitality, which we can all use!

243.   A single cup of juice will be equivalent to a much larger amount of actual vegetables or fruit, meaning one cup of juice can also be equal to make more servings on the food pyramid. For example, a single cup of carrot juice is equivalent to four cups of diced carrot!

244.   It's best to avoid juicing fruits and vegetables that have a low water content. Avocados and bananas, for example, are quite dense and don't have much water in them. They will clog up your juicer and you won't get much juice out of them. If you really want to include them, blend them first and then mix them with juices from other produce.

245.   Healthy juicing for kids can seem like a daunting task, leading people to only give them

fruit. Try carrot juice! Most kids absolutely adore it, and you can sneak many other vegetables in it without your child even noticing. You can also try having two or three fruit with wheatgrass, or protein powder, and the fruit will overwhelm the taste of anything you add.

246.   Sugar cane juice can help build your immune system, but chewing on the actual sugar cane can cause tooth decay. Instead, juice your sugar cane along with fruit, vegetables, and other healthy additives to get the most nutritious juices possible every single day. Juicing can taste great and help you stay healthy!

247.   There is no harm in juicing more than once a day as long as you're not just filling up on fruit juices. Fruit can be full of calories and sugar, so stick to vegetables as much as possible instead. If you want to add some sweetness to your veggie juice, try beets!

248.   A great juicing tip is to add a little bit of ginger to your juice. It will give your juice a little kick and it will also provide more nutritional benefits. Ginger has been used as medicine for many years and can be a great addition to any juice.

249.   A good juicing tip is to start with simple ingredients if you've never juiced before. A lot of people start juicing for the health benefits but if you start using really healthy ingredients right off the bat, you might find that the taste is just too bitter for you.

250.   If you've stored juice that you've made previously and are planning to drink it, put it out on the counter for at least 30 minutes to allow it to come to room temperature. Your body has a much easier time digesting foods which are not cold, so give your tummy a break!

251.   The pulp is beneficial to you since it has fibers and proteins that are not found in the juice. Juicy pulp packs a great deal of nutrients and much-needed fiber. Regardless of how much pulp you incorporate into your drinks, fiber will always be beneficial.

252.   Make sure that you always have what you need to make your juices. Always make sure that you have the food on hand where you can see it. Just like with keeping the juice machine visible, you need to keep the ingredients for your juices where you can see them. Otherwise, you could forget about them.

253.   Spread the word about your juicing habits. Talk to your friends, family members, acquaintances, co-workers, etc. everyday or week about your juicing and health plans. These people should be someone who will show interest and listen to you, along with being someone who will not negatively judge your healthy lifestyle.

254.   Be sure to take time out in between juicing batches to empty your bin. This is especially true when working with large quantities of fruits and vegetables. You need to stop the unit to empty the pulp bin as it fills up. The cutter or strainer should also be cleaned.

255.   If you are planning on juicing citrus fruits only, or primarily citrus fruits, consider purchasing a juicer that is designed just for citrus. Many juicers have trouble with the amount of pith in a citrus fruit. In addition, juicers with metal surfaces will become corroded over time after repeated exposure to citrus fruits.

256.   If you want your juice to be a certain texture or thickness, know that the softer the fruit is, the thicker the juice will be. The meat of softer fruits breaks up easily to make a thick nectar. Make

sure to add some harder fruits, such as apples and pears, for a thinner juice.

257.   Drink your juice soon after making it if you are looking to benefit from the health benefits. Juice starts to lose its benefits as soon as it comes out of the fruit or veggie. The longer you let it sit, the more it will lose, so go ahead and drink it as soon as possible to be able to let your body enjoy all the nutrients.

258.   Don't buy too many fruits and vegetables at a time if you're juicing. You might end up buying much more than you will use, and the extra food will decay and go to waste. Experiment with different amounts to see how much juice you drink a day, so you know how much produce you have to buy in advance.

259.   Juicing your vegetables is a great way to get the vitamins and minerals that are in them without having to actually take the time to prepare them. Many people simply do not have the time to prepare a gourmet meal each and every night. Juicing vegetables allows you to quickly and easily get the most nutrients out of them that you possibly can without spending a ton of time on them.

260.   The biggest key in juicing is curiosity. Wanting to try new foods, things you've never even heard of before, will make your journey more tasty and exciting! Explore international produce markets to find vegetables and fruit that could change your life forever. Look online to research what vitamins and nutrients they contain.

261.   Before you get started juicing, do a little bit of research on the different varieties of fruits and veggies available. Flavor mixing is always an issue, but the biggest issue is the nutritional value of various fruits and vegetables. Check to see which items contain which vitamins and minerals. You should strive to combine vegetables and fruits that offer a varying range of nutrients, and which can satisfy your daily nutritional needs. In addition to fueling your body with natural ingredients, you will also discover a world of unique and delicious flavors.

262.   Start juicing with the softer items in your ingredient list and then follow them up with the harder items. This will help clear the pulp from your machine to facilitate an easier clean up later. You want to work your machine in the easiest way possible to give it a long life.

263.   It's important when you are juicing to peel any non-organic produce and discard the peel. The greatest amount of pesticide is found on the skin of fruits and vegetables because it is sprayed on. While washing the produce will remove most of it, some of it will have become embedded in the skin.

264.   If you're feeling bloated or retaining water, put the right ingredients into your juice to help flush you out! Celery, cranberry, cucumber, and watermelon are all recommended to help your system let the water go, and they also hold many nutrients, vitamins, and other healthy benefits that are vital to good health.

265.   When it comes to juicing, one thing that you want to keep in mind is the fact that wheat grass is not only an extremely powerful tasting ingredient but it also provides many nutrients. This is important because you want to introduce this into your juices, but you need to be careful to not use too much due to its overpowering taste.

266.   If you're starting to feel old and tired, juicing can make you feel young again and give you back your energy. By juicing, you can gain nutrients able to sharpen your memory, alleviate joint

discomfort and halt the pace of cell death resulting from free radicals.

267.   When it comes to juicing, one thing that you want to keep in mind is the fact that you do not need to depend on multivitamins or other supplements as much when using your juicer on a regular basis. This is beneficial because it will help you financially and give you a fun and tasty way to obtain the same nutrients.

268.   Choose a variety of vegetables to put in your juicer, based on their nutritional value. If their flavor isn't appealing to you, add some other ingredient to improve the flavor. This will provide your body with nutrients that you might have been missing out on otherwise. Add apple or lemon juice to cover up a taste you do not like.

269.   If you'd like to add protein supplements to your juice, wait a few days before you start. Your system will be getting used to the juice (which is easy as it's half-way digested by the time it gets to your stomach!) and flushing out toxins, so give it a chance to catch up first.

270.   A great juicing tip is to not overdo it if you're relatively new to juicing. Our bodies need time to

adjust to changes. If you start drinking super healthy green juices, you might find yourself making several trips to the bathroom every day. Moderation is the key when it comes to juicing.

271.   At the beginning of a juicing program, make juices out of fruits that you already enjoy eating. This will ensure that you enjoy the juice while still receiving some health benefits. If you start juicing using fruits you've never tried before, you may not like the juice and you're unlikely to continue making them, meaning you won't gain any benefits.

272.   If you are juicing greens, try rolling them into a ball first. Using the ball method is much more efficient for your juicer to handle than just trying to send your greens in there in their normal leafy state. Keep your juicing quick and efficient for optimum results.

273.   If you don't have time to juice in the morning, you can make juice on the weekend and drink it throughout the week. The truth is that the vitamins and other nutrients in the drink will break up as time passes, but it's better to drink homemade juice, than nothing at all!

274.   While juicing add some fish oil or cod liver oil. These two types of oils will help with the absorption of vitamin K. The fats from fish oil are very beneficial for health and gives you the right amount and the right kinds of fat needed for vitamin K absorption.

275.   Buying a masticating juicer will allow the juice you make to have it's nutrients break down much slower, meaning you can take your time in drinking it or even store it for a while. It will also leave as much of the natural nutrients intact as possible, giving you the most healthy juice to drink.

276.   Drinking juice is one of the best ways to get the nutrients and enzymes your body needs. So do you buy bottled juice or make your own juice? Making your own juice promises the freshest taste possible as well as giving you the means to create flavorful combinations.

277.   When it comes to juicing, one thing that you want to keep in mind is to be sure that you stay away from certain types of dry or squishy products when buying your ingredients. This is important because certain fruits and vegetables such as bananas and squash are just simply not suited for juicing.

278.	When it comes to juicing, one thing that you want to keep in mind is to make sure that you have space set aside in your kitchen for your juicing machine and for the preparation of your ingredients. This is important so that you are efficient and so that you are motivated to make juice as often as possible. Having to clean clutter out of the way would just be a deterrent.

279.	The best time to juice is first thing in the morning when you have an empty stomach. Your body can fully digest and assimilate the juice because there will be nothing else for it to compete with. Within 30 minutes the nutrients will be fully absorbed into the blood stream.

280.	When it comes to juicing, one thing that you want to keep in mind is the fact that many fruits and vegetables have the most amount of nutrients either in the skins or directly beneath them. This is important to consider when deciding whether or not to peel your ingredients.

281.	Drink your juice as quickly as possible. In order to get the best juice, it is very important to note that nutrients from the juice are lost once the juice is made. If you take a long time to drink it, you'll be getting fewer of the benefits of the beverage. Therefore, it's recommended to consume juice as soon as possible.

282.   Juicing is not the miracle cure for everything that ails you! It is important that juicing is just a part of your new healthy lifestyle, from eating a healthy diet full of raw foods to exercising as often as possible. Drinking homemade juice will help boost your energy, giving you the drive to get active!

283.   Fresh juice is a wonderful source of many vitamins and minerals. Not only does juicing provide you with energy, but it can help give you the drive to exercise and gain muscle. If your exercise routine is on the harder side, opt for vegetables and fruits that replenish electrolytes after your workout, and whey protein powder can be added to help rebuild muscle fibers.

284.   In regards to juicing, it is important to consider how much of a benefit certain ingredients such as carrots will provide to your skin care. Carrots are one of the best ways to obtain vitamin A, which is known to cut back on the production of your body's natural oils. It will also help in the production of new and healthy skin cells.

285.   Detoxing the colon is fun and easy by juicing! Apples and lemons are an excellent choice for a detox recipe as they both are known to help cleanse the colon. You can also include beets, carrots, celery, ginger, and radishes. Almost any juice you make will help to heal your body, so feel free to use whatever items you really enjoy.

286.   When using fruits to create your juice, it is important to remove seeds and pits, if there are any. For example, you must remove pits from peaches and seeds from apples. Adding these items can quickly deteriorate the quality of the blades in the juicer and possibly, even break the juicer. Furthermore, certain seeds like apple seeds can be dangerous because they contain trace amounts of cyanide.

287.   Peel citrus fruits before you put them in your juicer. The thick peels of citrus fruits will make your juice taste unpleasant, provide no real health benefit, and can even be harmful. The greatest benefit from citrus fruits comes from the white pith just below the peel, so be sure to retain that when juicing.

288.   To eliminate the pulp from your home made juice, use a cheesecloth or coffee filter to strain

the pulp out. If you choose to remove the pulp from your juice remember that you are also removing many vitamins and minerals. For the healthiest juice, drink it with pulp and all.

289.   When preparing for a juice diet, make sure to stock a LOT of fresh fruits and vegetables! On average, it takes 4.4 pounds of raw fruits and vegetables to make just a single quart of juice, so you'll need lots. Also make sure to get a large variety of ingredients so that you don't get bored with the same old juice.

290.   Keep the juicer on your kitchen counter in plain sight. This constant visual reminder will help you take advantage of juicing more often. It will be a simple matter to drop in a few fruits and veggies and make fresh healthy juice every day.

291.   Find a juicing community online and sign up to learn more about what others have tried. They'll have tons of recipe ideas, warnings about things they tried and failed, and support for you when you're feeling overwhelmed. They will also have money-saving tips and tricks that you might not have thought of before!

292.   Let color be your guide for variety. You will want to keep your juicing varied so as to not get

bored with it. Incorporate a variety of colors in your fruits and vegetables as a sort of juicing palette from which to create. Just remember to know the nutrient content from each source and enjoy the rainbow.

293.   When juicing with leafy greens such as kale or chard, consider adding cucumber to balance out the flavors. Cucumbers also have a ton of nutrients and vitamins in them which are super healthy for you, so they're a great addition to any juice. Throw in a fruit for sweetness and you'll have one heck of a nutritious but tasty drink!

294.   When it comes to juicing, one thing that you want to keep in mind is that you will want to make sure that you purchase all of your fruits and vegetables from local farmers markets. Local farmers markets often will have a greater selection and lower prices than normal grocery stores.

295.   By juicing fruits and vegetables you are basically pre-digesting it so that your stomach will have a far easier time passing the nutrients directly from the juice itself to your cells. This will provide an almost immediate boost to your energy levels, your health, and your overall sense of well being.

296.   When it comes to juicing, one thing that you want to keep in mind is the fact that wheat grass is not only an extremely powerful tasting ingredient but it also provides many nutrients. This is important because you want to introduce this into your juices, but you need to be careful to not use too much due to its overpowering taste.

297.   In order to get the most out of your juice it is good to get the right kind of juicer. Some juice extractors generate unwanted heat during the operation and tend to deal damage to the delicate structure of the juice. This destroys the nutrients that are in the juice.

298.   A major benefit of juicing is the high volume of healthy nutrients that are made easily available. In order to maximize those nutrients, the base of the juice should be made from vegetables like spinach, kale, chard or broccoli. By using these vegetables you will achieve the maximum health benefits including a low amount of sugar, which is usually a dominant ingredient in store-bought juices.

299.   In regards to juicing, it is important to consider the fact that juices can actually work to

prevent cancer in your body. The benefit from this is obvious and it does so through the maintenance of proper pH levels. Many types of produce also work to rid the body of toxins.

300.   Store dark, leafy vegetables in tightly-sealed plastic bags to keep them fresh until it's time to juice. Before bagging the vegetables, rinse them thoroughly and use a towel to dry them off.

301.   You can combat constipation by juicing vegetables such as cabbage, fennel, beetroot, papaya, parsnips and lettuce. If constipation is a recurring issue, drinking juices regularly will help you regulate your system.

302.   When using juicing as part of your weight loss program, make sure you're doing it at a time that works best for you. If you find you're rushing or stressed while creating your juices then you're likely to quit. Work it into your life as best you can, so if you can only do it every other day, it's better than nothing!

303.   A good juicing tip is to consider not juicing if you're pregnant. The reason you shouldn't juice if you're pregnant is because your child might be born with a vitamin C deficiency. This

can happen because their vitamin C intake will drop severely as soon as they are born.

304.   Juice is best consumed fresh. Trying to save juice for more than an hour or so will reduce the amount of active nutrients in the drink and let the drink settle too. Make your juice and drink it right away. If you want to save some for a family member who will be drinking it shortly that is fine, otherwise you will want to make it fresh for them later.

305.   Drink your juice on an empty stomach, such as first thing in the morning or about half an hour before a meal. This allows your system to better absorb the nutrients in your juice, without the interference of other foods. Juice drunk on an empty stomach can enter your system in as quickly as thirty minutes.

306.   Think of the juice as your whole meal. When you find out how much food goes into a glass of juice after preparing it several times, you will understand why this is so. Treating juice as a meal replacement allows your body to quickly absorb nutrients into your bloodstream.

307.   To get more variety in taste from your juicer, mix up the varieties of fruits and vegetables you

put in your juicer and the variety of flavors will grow significantly. Try mixing orange, banana and pineapple for a tasty tropical treat or mix grape and cranberry for more antioxidants. These home made juices are healthier and easier to make then those sugar-filled, store bought juices.

308.   The best rule for getting into juicing is that the juicer should be out and visible all the time. This will remind you to use it, and also make it easier to use so you don't skip it because you don't want to lug it out. Keeping it in sight will also keep it in mind.

309.   There are a million-and-one recipes of items to include in your juicer. You can try a combination like apple with carrot and ginger, or celery and pear. My favorites are apple with lemon and pear, apple with cinnamon and honey, and, my daughter's favorite, banana with mango and orange. Try new ideas to find your own favorites!

310.   The best time to fire up your juicer is a half hour before any meal. Drink the fresh juice on an empty stomach. Drinking juice on an empty stomach is helpful to absorb the most nutrients quickly and effectively. Fruit juices should be

consumed in the mornings because digestive energy is the lowest in the mornings.

311. Drinking juice is one of the best ways to get the nutrients and enzymes your body needs. So do you buy bottled juice or make your own juice? Making your own juice promises the freshest taste possible as well as giving you the means to create flavorful combinations.

312. To improve your general health quickly and easily, drink green juices. These are fresh juices made from leafy green vegetables. To improve the flavor and add a variety of nutrients, include such fruits and oranges and bananas. These juices are quick to make, taste great, and will give you energy that lasts for hours.

313. When it comes to juicing, one thing that you want to keep in mind is the fact that despite the time and money that you are losing by making your own juice, you will find that it most likely tastes better than store bought juice. This is important to give you a good reason to keep on juicing and influence others to do the same.

314. It's always better to use organic fruit when making juices, but since they are pricy, you can't always get organic fruit. When using non-organic

produce, there might be harmful pesticides that you don't want to put into your drinks. So, make sure you peel the fruits so you don't ingest the pesticides.

315.   When it comes to juicing, one thing that you want to keep in mind is the amount of fruits and vegetables you are purchasing in relation to the amount of juice that you wish to produce. A good rule of thumb is that one cup of juice will result from approximately a pound of product.

316.   If you'd like to add protein supplements to your juice, wait a few days before you start. Your system will be getting used to the juice (which is easy as it's half-way digested by the time it gets to your stomach!) and flushing out toxins, so give it a chance to catch up first.

317.   Jerusalem artichokes are an excellent addition to the juice you make as they will kill any craving your sweet tooth throws at you! They aren't the most flavorful food, though, so add other items like lemon juice and carrot to make a drink that you'll enjoy and will keep you healthy.

318.	Serve your juice quickly after you prepared it. Ideally you will drink your juice as soon as you make it.

319.	Educate yourself about the number of fruits and vegetables that are available for purchase. A lot of people aren't aware of the selection of vegetables and fruits that are available to you. Buy something you've never tried before every time you go food shopping. This stops you from getting bored with juicing, as you might if you drank the same type of juice every day.

320.	Do not make the same juice blend every day. You have a juicer, so get creative. You will gain the best benefits from drinking different fruits and vegetables every day, not drinking many in the same juice. Trying different juices everyday is more exciting and allows you to get creative.

321.	When you are using green, leafy vegetables, like spinach or cabbage, for an extra-healthy juice, roll the leaves together in a ball and add them to the juicer in that form. Making the leaves into a fruit-like shape will help make better juice than throwing in a handful of leaves.